taking chemo on the chin

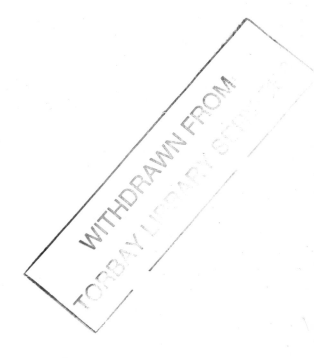

KCC

taking chemo on the chin

simple advice from the other side of treatment

Richard Armitt

A helpful, honest and humorous look at the treatment of
cancer, from the point of view of the author, a survivor.

First published in New Zealand by Koru Cottage Consulting Ltd, 2009

www.koru-cottage.com

disclaimer

The opinions and experiences contained in this work are personally related to the author, his chemotherapy regime and his reactions to treatment of his disease.

Printed by Publishing Press Ltd, Auckland

ISBN: 978-0-473-14595-8

dedication

To my darling Sophie, for sitting up front in our rollercoaster
love you for sharing my world my Princess of Bubbles

Also thanks to family and friends that helped us through
some trying times, especially Mum and Dad for being there.

Mr. Gavin Wall for his eternal humour, love of action figures
and being Bruce to my Clark.

Not forgetting the Doctors and team at WDHB in Auckland
– thank you for fixing me.

Finally, a nod to the community and team at
www.buttonmasher.co.nz for good times online

Introduction

I used to be indestructible.

I was a man of steel.

Or so I thought.

I was reasonably fit, reasonably healthy, and reasonably active; then all that changed overnight.

Discovering my lymphoma in August 2006 led to six months of physical and psychological hardship, fortunately for us things turned out well and two years later I am feeling mostly good as new.

After the operation, consultations, procedures and the three months of fortnightly outpatient R-CHOP chemotherapy, I had experienced things I never dreamt would come my way.

Now that my superhero days are behind me, I would like to share some thoughts and tips to help whoever else may be wandering this long and well trodden road.

Life is a challenging journey and sometimes we get thrown a curveball that seems to obliterate everything and anything that was important to us five minutes before, the fact is that time moves us on and life always finds a way to regain control.

Physical aspects of your life - like strength, stamina and energy become critical factors that need constant nurturing and should never be taken for granted.

If you are a patient I want to give you this information to help you in an informal and non-clinical way, offering tips, and honest experience that may make you feel better prepared for the battle ahead.

Or you might be supporting a friend or loved one through treatment; hopefully this book will give you an insight into the experience ahead and also shed some light on what may pass through your minds over the coming months.

I was not prepared for the moment that I sat in a doctor's consultation room and listen to him tell me that I had cancer. I was shocked, then I panicked and finally I found myself in a vacuum.

I doubted myself, blamed myself and looked for reason where there were none.

I expected answers to questions I could not bring myself to ask.

Let's clear a couple of questions up from the start:

"What did I do wrong?"

There is no right or wrong, and it won't change anything.

"When did it begin?"

A date may help give you perspective, but it won't change anything.

"Why did it happen to me?"

Why does it happen to anybody? And it still won't change anything.

Sophie's page

The day we found out Richard had lymphoma; we were both in utter shock. You never believe it's going to happen to you or your loved one.

I have learned from this that you can't be super strong all the time, it puts a lot of pressure on yourself and maybe people around you. Have a good cry or shout if you want to.

Richard has been amazing and just got on with his treatment and recovery. Nothing fancy, just a daily juice, he listened to his body regarding rest and appetite, although gravy was off the menu for a while.

We complemented each other by being supportive when the other of us was not feeling strong.

My advice is to get support and help for yourself as well, someone you can talk to about your fears. Be kind to yourselves and remember nobody knows what is around the corner in life.

Sophie x x x

taking chemo on the chin

So, you've been diagnosed with cancer, Should you have gone to the doctor sooner?

A lot of cancer symptoms can be matched to more common afflictions and it is unusual for them all to be picked out in the early stages. Unless you have been ignoring a sizable lump for a couple of months you probably went to the doctor as soon as you discovered it, give or take the normal period of panic and doubt.

The key thing to remember is that now you are in the health system there are caring professionals involved that want to make you well again.

It's not all about you

This was something of a motto for us.

Being really sick allows you to feel pretty down, but spare a thought for the people around you who are also being affected.

In any relationship both sides have to pull together and help each other through their respective dips, be aware of how partners or friends may be feeling.

Remember that supporting and nurturing are nicer when shared.

Do I have a big 'Keep Away' sign to carry around with me?

It might feel like it.

Inside your bubble the world starts to look different and you question how people look at you, and whether or not they want to acknowledge you.

Some people prefer sandwich boards.

How do I talk to people?

I take my time.

Coming out with bad news is difficult, and having to judge uncomfortable reactions around you can be difficult.

For example in a workplace you might be surprised by the people who are sympathetic and genuinely concerned as opposed to the people that may be closer to you, but treat you like a pariah to hide their own fears.

Remember it's their bag of rocks and they can deal with it themselves.

It's *your* disease now

I remember being sat in front of somebody that kept telling me about *my* disease, which was uncomfortable.

I wasn't in denial that's for definite, but I was taking it in slowly, understanding things my way. So when I was suddenly labeled with this life threatening insult that I did not consider mine, I now felt that it was time for a reality check.

When we want something for ourselves, we go out and get it, a television or some furniture maybe, but not cancer.

At the end of the day, the sooner you understand that you have it, and the disease is now yours. Then the sooner you can start to move on and get positive about the treatment.

Research and read as much POSITIVE information as you can

The internet can be a wonderful thing, a bottomless fountain of knowledge that covers many wonderful subjects.

The trick and focus of any research exercise is to keep aiming for positive information, find the good stories, research the new developments in treatment, look for energizing diet advice, and above all keep building a positive attitude.

Use search engines wisely, using words like 'positive', 'success', and 'recovery'. You will be surprised at the good stuff and will not get dragged down by the negative side of your situation.

Do not believe all you read online, especially if you have to pay for it

Generally good advice and research pays dividends if it's free, although for all the genuine people out there that want to help and advise you there are plenty of profiteers that will want your credit card details first.

Come to terms with your disease and understand it as best as you can. This will help you to sort the wheat from the chaff, but remember that the World Wide Web is like a tomato – it's better with a pinch of salt.

Stop wishing your problem onto others, even if they are more deserving

There is always somebody more deserving:

The unfit guy eating a pie at the bus stop

The bleary-eyed wife beater down the street

The old lady that smokes thirty cigarettes a day

Wishing your disease onto somebody that you consider 'should' have caught it isn't good for you, it is momentarily distracting, but it won't help you achieve anything.

Don't feel ashamed or alone, it's a natural reaction that every survivor I've met admits too.

You just have to focus on dealing with it, now.

Get your colours into you;
take on board Anti-oxidants
and plenty of them

Mainly fruit and vegetables — that five a day mix of natural food has never been more important, there are many schools of thought regarding which will be of the most benefit.

My advice is don't force yourself to eat it if you don't like it.

There is a huge range of colourful food to choose from that can be eaten raw or cooked. There will be choices that you will enjoy.

Apples, carrots, oranges, grapefruit, prunes, peppers, and tomatoes the list goes on and on.

And don't ignore the other super foods — nuts may not be colourful, but they are full of good stuff too.

Daily juicing - If you don't enjoy eating fruits and vegetables drink them instead

A great way to keep up your anti-oxidant intake and a good routine to get into, a refreshing fruit cocktail each morning can give you a great energy boost and will be laden with vitamins that you might normally be missing out on.

My favorite way to start the day is a juice consisting of:

- 2 carrots
- 2 apples
- 2 oranges
- 1 healthy nugget of ginger

Apart from being tasty, they are packed full of anti oxidants, a dose of anti-inflammatory properties and plenty of natural goodness.

It will also keep your mouth fresh when dry.

Don't forget the ice.

Ensure that you leave every consultation appointment satisfied

This can be a bewildering time, lurching from one specialist appointment to another riding a physical and emotional rollercoaster.

Your clinical appointments are your window of opportunity to gain as much new knowledge as you can. This is where the real information should come from.

Keep asking questions and don't be afraid to look or feel silly, you have a right to completely understand what is happening to you.

Don't forget that you are new to this and it takes time for people to adjust and learn new things.

Understanding your treatment cycle

You need to feel as in control of your situation as much as you possibly can. Once you have been sat down and shown your array of medicines and/or injections you need to be super practical.

Lay it out in a diary or on a calendar, scheduled treatment days, appointments, scans, even a rolling chart for tablet taking.

Whether you like to tick things off or not, it will give you an overview of the process; a holistic view that will help you put the goal into perspective.

Keep the end in mind, keep a positive focus, and keep getting closer to the end of the treatment.

Sweating in the dread of night

Night sweats are an experience.

They might start slowly and be mistaken for a stuffy night or the result of spicy food, but once they get going you really know about it.

I am by nature a hot person and no stranger to sweating, but I was not prepared for the drenching effect of a solid night sweat. Even sleeping on towels was limited in its effectiveness, as I would regularly wake up shortly after midnight literally swimming.

It can leave you feeling dirty and dreading the night. There is a bright side though, as treatment progresses and symptoms begin to recede so do the sweats.

Plan some fun for you

No need to curl up in a ball just yet, make sure you remember what you like to do and have some fun.

Make sure that there is stuff on that calendar that has nothing to do with treatment and being sick, events or activities that will make you smile will be enough.

Do something creative, catch up with friends, enjoy a quiet coffee in the presence of strangers who don't know you as the sick person, the list can be endless.

If you look hard enough you will see the sign as you leave the hospital: "The fun doesn't stop here".

Plan some fun for those closest to you

Nearly everybody has access to support, from their nearest and dearest; these people are suffering with you every step of the way. They see you change physically in appearance, and how you cope with a flight of steps. They may also be ferrying you around to your appointments or helping you with injections.

You could be suffering, but never forget your loved ones suffer for you too; make some time for them, plan to do something enjoyable with them that you can both treasure, or simply spoil them.

Come up with something, as far from sickness as possible; the lighter the better. It doesn't have to be extravagant or life changing; a simple picnic in the park can feel as special as a night at the Ritz.

Side effects, a way of life

The treatment is hard on your body and it will suffer. Along with that difficulty you will also receive a mixed bag of side effects.

On average side effects can vary vastly from patient to patient depending entirely on how you react to your treatment, I will deal with some of the major side effects separately; losing your hair, for example, is pretty much a safe bet.

Side effects will be present during and after your treatment, but, the thing to remember is that they are there for good reason.

So whether you develop blisters on your feet, have bouts of insomnia, can't keep food down or have a mouth full of ulcers, keep a focus on your recovery and come through your treatment stronger for it.

Shedding hair, is the most obvious and stereotypical sign of treatment

What they didn't tell you is that it does actually hurt.

It will happen, even if not straight away; but it will happen and the degree of severity of hair loss will vary from patient to patient.

Your hair may be dying and you hair will be loose, but they will not have let go just yet. You will simply turn over in bed one day and feel a scattering of pinpricks over your scalp as they are gently tugged out; it's an irritating pain that serves to remind you of what is happening.

Hair loss is something of a watershed; mentally it's akin to the point of no return on a journey. It's the point where you step over from being a sick person to a chemo patient in strangers' eyes.

Blisters

According to my medical team, blisters are not common, but the world wide web of wonders will inform you otherwise.

I consider if you have chemicals in your body that are destroying your soft cell structure then they will get to your skin at some stage. From somewhere around the halfway treatment point my feet developed a fair covering of blisters, painful to walk on and nasty to deal with. When every step racks you with sharp and salty pains you can get quite down quite quickly.

Luckily I had some previous blister experience to draw from after completing some long distance walks. If it hurts, your body is doing its job telling you about it, and, even though you don't want to walk on them you can, and will.

Advice is only a short phone call away

One of the great things about the medical system is the back-up and support that is available. While the front line surgeons and doctors deal with the major issues, there are dedicated people ready and willing to ferret out answers to those burning questions.

Nurses, patient specialists and dedicated support workers are there in some form, ready to help and working for you.

They can help with enquiries and make positive suggestions, or simply put a worried patient at ease with their knowledge and experience.

Find out who is available, get their number, don't be afraid to use it and remember that you will never be wasting their time.

Nail Beds

Once my fingernails and tips became sensitive I was truly amazed at how often I bashed my fingers each day without noticing.

At its worst this side effect was like hitting my finger tips with a hammer every time I went to pick up or touch something and missed. Wrap them up, and take care when using your hands.

Nail beds will be affected by the treatment, nails will lift and some may even fall off.

They will grow back.

Apart from a surgery scar, my toe nails were the last physical part of me to return to normal.

It just takes time.

Become a Food Monster

your appetite can be
disrupted by your
treatment

One aspect of my approach to my illness which has amazed people is the way I generally coped with food.

I kept my body fuelled up; I listened to what it wanted and gave it exactly that. I stocked up on good healthy energy giving foods. A weekend was not complete without a spicy Thai Green Curry and my lunchtimes were not complete without a foot long Subway.

It's no good just wasting away. Your body needs a ton of energy to fuel it for the battle it's fighting on your behalf.

Don't be afraid of putting on weight, firstly there are worse things that can happen, secondly the medication, treatment and disease will do a pretty good job of stopping that happening.

Taste and Smell

Both taste and smell can be subjective and certainly depend on the individual and their preferences.

Taste and smell are also linked very closely to memories, so a smell that turns your stomach while you are ill may well stay with you for some time.

Even now I gag at the thought of the hospital soup. On Friday (treatment day) it was vegetable and the memory still flares my nostrils and turns my stomach.

You will learn to avoid certain smells and tastes because of their affect on you, it's normal and understandable, besides you may become a healthier person for the sake of it.

Acid Reflux

Your body is suffering and yet your system will be bombarded with a host of unnatural things, chemicals and poisons that are design to kill your most vulnerable cells.

This process will leave many scars, it's to be expected.

After experiencing many periods where I could not even lie flat for the stomach acid rising, I thought, this really is worth a mention.

There will be uncomfortable times so make sure you get some medication. It is there for the asking and will help you recover.

A burning gullet is most unpleasant especially when you are feeling low; plain and calming foods will help ease the discomfort.

Black Gold

I enjoyed getting into the habit of enjoying a Guinness.

At first the thick, black beer is an acquired taste, and then it became a real treat as the smooth nutty liquid slipped down.

There is another terrific reason too; it's like an injection of liquid iron, eat a ton of spinach if you want to, but I believe my blood fared well on a daily can of the black stuff.

Treatment Day

Have a good breakfast before you go to treatment.

Do get used to wheeling yourself to the toilet with your drip attached to you; it's going to happen a lot so there's no point in being shy.

After a couple of chemo sessions you will know what to take with you to feel comfortable. Reading and writing may be difficult, wearing big comfy socks and snoozing is not.

In the evening when you are ready to eat, something plain and simple like a boiled egg and toast soldiers may be comforting.

Depending on how you react to chemo you may not sleep for the first night at least, so get a taste for late night TV.

Mmmm, Barley Sugars

Rediscover the boiled sweets of the old days, sucking on a Barley Sugar can loosen up that dry mouth and deliver a nice hit of sugar too.

From a personal perspective Pear Drops were too acidic and Mints have a short term effect, where as the soothing taste of a Barley Sugar can linger and re-invigorate your palette.

Medication

Medication continues on from treatment day. You will have a tough regime of tablets to swallow, from the effective anti-nausea tablets to kidney saving combinations.

During each cycle you will have to take certain tablets on certain days — believe me by the end of the cycle you will have had enough of them.

A shadow on my shoulder

Your world will be the same only different.

Everybody has dark days. The trick is learning to live with the shadow of fear, by accepting its presence and getting on with your life.

When you have faced your darkest fears, there will be times when you forget about them. And there will be days when your fears fill the room behind you.

Believe me there will be days when you realize you haven't thought about your fears at all. Strangely you may even feel guilty, the best bet is to make sure those shadow free days outweigh the dark days.

Self injecting

Modern treatments open up all sorts of experiences and one of the most alien is to stab your skin with a needle.

The first time I did it, I whacked the needle in after three tries. Looked at the needle embedded in my skin for a second then yanked it out again. It took another five minutes to get it back in.

Just be patient and get used to the prick, timing is important; best to pick a time that won't clash with other activities.

Just remember that, one day; you will be able to forget all about them.

I let my injection reminder alarm run for a few days extra, enjoying turning it off and not reaching for the pack of syringes.

Panic and Worry

These two emotions make terrific bedfellows; even when everything is going well one stray thought, ache or pain can bring on the double act of panic and worry.

Rule 1: It's perfectly normal to experience panic when you think you are in trouble again. Just take a deep breath and rationalize your fear. Question your reason for panic; validate it against the treatment regime and your noted progress so far.

Rule 2: Your mind can play tricks on you. In your current situation you need to be positive, stay focused on healing and even the most responsive patients can find themselves in a dark and gloomy place scared about the future.

Rationalize, focus and stay positive.

Habitual Palpating

As humans we seek knowledge and validation, especially when our health is at risk. Before, during and after treatment you will most likely spend plenty of time feeling for signs of recovery or relapse.

With a disease that manifests in physical terms it's completely natural to want to be feeling for signs, checking their progress and stability.

You have to try. I know it is hard I know, but you have to try to stop feeling for trouble. Whether driving, in the shower, in bed, in the office or in public.

It may be best to try to restrict your personal palpating to limited sessions, maybe every other day at first then move on to weekly.

Follow up appointments

When necessary appointments appear on the horizon you will start to worry about your check up. By the day you get to the hospital you may be stressed and fretting enough to make yourself feel sick.

Make the most of the appointment to ask questions about your progress, check out those bumps and scars that you have been feeling for the last few months, listen to the expert's opinion.

After the appointment you will feel relieved and glad to have gotten it under your belt.

Then after a natural rest period you will start to worry about the next appointment.

Promise yourself that one day you will go to a check up without stressing; now that will be a good day.

The first day chemo's over

What should I do now?

Get on with my life, go on holiday, get that new job, rest, recover, and revel in your time.

How will I feel?

Relieved at least for a while, then the worry will probably set in. I try not to let it gnaw away at my mind.

Will it change me?

Probably not in the Hollywood sense that I might have imagined, but I feel that my outlook may be stronger, and I am able to deal with your regular life with more confidence.

This is a time for you to really look forward to a point that is beyond the cycle of treatment you have just endured.

A lifetime of milestones:

this week becomes a month

that month becomes 6 months

6 months becomes a year

that year becomes 2 years

There will come a time when you stop worrying about your next scan and or appointment, or at least you will worry less than you are right now. The treatment system still has your back, even if in your absence, checking your blood tests and scheduling your appointments. The trick is to blend these aftercare milestones into a timeline of your own that incorporates other personal goals.

A holiday is a milestone.

Participating in a sponsored event for charity is a milestone.

Feeling strong enough to make a bungee jump, proves you now know how to live on the edge. Depending on the jumper this is also a milestone.

Keep on talking and don't mind your mouth

Some people find it hard to talk; some people just clam up to protect themselves.

You are in the best position to talk about yourself, your feelings, and your experiences so do not be afraid to discuss them all.

People may not react very well, they may even become upset, but this is your life in the balance and if something needs to be said then get it out there, you are coping and the more you talk the easier it will become.

Keep venting your worries – don't be a pressure cooker

Everybody needs to let off steam occasionally, especially you.

If you find that your fears and niggling worries are building up inside you then you will become a boiling pot of negative energy and stress.

Don't hold onto your fears, let off a little steam and the pressure will ease, there may be tears of joy, relief or sadness but you will feel better.

Also remember that sharing these feelings with your support person will allow them to vent too, there is nothing worse than watching somebody you love suffer in silence, always talk it out.

Crawl

before

walking

before

running

Recovery can be a slow and challenging process; personal fitness depends on you and your body working together

Don't expect to run marathons two months after completing your course it takes serious time to repair you, eat well, listen to your body and be mindful of your fragility.

Once you are past the treatment and beginning to feel well it can be easy to set yourself back with over confidence, marching up a giant sand dune with rock bottom energy took all my strength and was an achievement, but I know I should have sat it out. When I got to the top my heart was pounding out of my chest, I had legs like jelly and my breathing was painfully ragged, but I did it and the ride down on a boogie board was terrific.

Take your time, get fit gracefully, finish work early if you are tired and be proud of how far you've come each day.

Everything always happens

for a reason

It's ugly and nasty and depressing, but hey there must be some reason for a plan like this.

Another lifetime philosophy for me, 'Everything does happen for a reason', call it fate, kismet or some crazy gods grand design. I don't care why, but it helps things make sense.

I remember being sat on a bed talking to my Mother on the other side of the world and telling her how I felt normal, how everything we were going through didn't seem unnatural.

The sooner you embrace the fact that it's happening and adjust to dealing with the cause and effect of the treatment, the sooner you can move on.

Getting used to needles

Needles, lots of needles, between the blood tests and self injected medication you will have your fill.

If you are the kind of person that doesn't like needles you will have to get used to them, they do get easier to bear.

The lucky ones that get to experience a bone marrow aspiration will tell you that the needles get easier as the treatment progresses, because that procedure is one of the first, biggest and singularly most painful experiences on the curriculum.

Don't accept crap from anybody

People around you may find it hard to cope and sometimes that will be delivered via sarcastic or awkward comments.

Like the idiot that choose to point out my comfortable shoes and make a joke of my supposed jogging to work, when the reason for my shoes was coping with blistered and painful feet. This attitude was especially offensive at a time when I could not even climb a single flight of stairs without stopping to rest and catch my breath.

I was not amused and explained that frankly and in full.

Like an animal, when you are down and injured and backed into a corner you are entitled to respond accordingly.

You have your own problems, let them deal with theirs.

Know your gown, before you strip

Left alone in a hospital changing room and presented with a strange garment.

My advice is to work out exactly how a gown works before you take your clothes off, understand where to put your arms and which side is the front.

I have spent some anxious semi-naked moments behind a fluttering curtain as nurses kept asking if I was ready.

Think ahead and keep as relaxed as possible.

You are not a victim

You are a survivor.

It's a disease not a vendetta and if the cause was apparent we would be spending time not catching it.

The human spirit is a great thing that sets us apart from the animal kingdom, we learn to deal with our situation and develop strategy to cope with adversity.

Be positive, win the war and be battle scarred survivor.

Getting used to paranoia

As time goes on the paranoia lessens, but when it hits it hits you hard.

Months from now you may casually touch your body and feel something is out of place; you may just feel under the weather or wake up with a cold sweat in the night.

Panic will swamp you and the world will go quiet, you can learn to see the symptoms of the paranoia as they rise and aim to put a lid on them. Rationalize your fear, look at the symptoms objectively – are they really symptoms? And are they really more than coincidence?

Try to remind yourself that this feeling will be gone in a week or so and you will feel as well as you did before you got the fear.

Some days are better than others

Some days have bouncers that won't let you in.

Nobody can be ultra positive every minute of every day especially when you are vulnerable.

The lesson is to see the day for what it is, if you can't face it stay under the duvet, and ignore that black dog. Work can wait and a routine will continue tomorrow, that's why it's called a routine.

You are not just feeling a bit down you are surviving something terrible and the toll it takes can be expensive? Sometimes you need to say no to spending energy on a bad day. Invest in yourself.

Build up some positive reserve today and use that to make tomorrow better.

Keep some aspect of a normal routine

Living with the disease and coping with the treatment is bewildering, without even considering the implications that haunt you every day.

Keep a slice of normality in your routine, try to maintain some work even if it's part-time, see friends, do the shopping or go to the movies.

It can be far too easy to hide away like a prisoner in your own home, get outside and have some things to look forward to.

The treatment is energy sapping and emotionally draining, but keeping a few normal adventures alive can be energy giving rather than letting it drain away in front of the TV.

Enjoy the simple things

The colours of the sky, the wind in the grass, and the laughter of a loved one - are they clichés?

Perhaps they are, but there are many wonderfully simple things in life that we miss out on and ignore; this is not a lesson in how to be a better person.

Remind yourself that 'It's not all about you'. There are many facets of life all around you that can lighten your day and lift your mood, so don't wallow in the dark days.

Get out there and enjoy the simple things.

Rest, rest, rest

By the end of your treatment cycle your body is depleted and you will be listless, you will have the immunity of a newborn.

This is a dangerous time; often the relief of finishing a treatment cycle brings down your natural defenses leaving you open to regular illness.

Build some energy by resting.

Recovery takes time and each day will have a different effect on you, draining you. Build yourself back up slowly; find some respect for your new and improved body.

Listen to your inner voice, allow it some leeway, and if it tells you to go to bed early, just do it.

Be proud of your progress

You are amazing, your body is amazing and the very fact that medical professionals can fix you at a cellular level is beyond comprehension.

Revel in your successes and grow stronger from disappointments.

Your treatment is affecting your body at a cellular level, and when it is over you will have been reset, your immune system will be virgin territory and will need supporting, eat well and take supplements to stave off any infection.

Don't push it, be proud of your progress and build on it gradually.

Be wary of statistics

Sometimes measuring things in percentage terms can be beneficial, but it can also be misleading.

A 75% chance of recovery or a 1 in 4 possibility of not recovering, which would you prefer to be told?

Statistics can make us feel better about the outlook we have in one breath and bleak in the next.

Try and not read too much in to them.

Use your imagination

I have always been a fan of my own imagination; it's a great way to waste time, watching your own home movies on the inside of your head.

Something I liked to do, especially when lying in the dark keeping the dark thoughts away was by using my imagination to picture my healing.

Like a microscopic army of robots that came with my chemo, seeking out destroying the alien invaders, some of those battles were truly magnificent.

Stress can make you ill, laughter can help you heal, and it stands to reason that thinking about how you are getting better can add to your recovery.

Positive Images

Picture yourself:

...as strong as a superhero and fitter than an Olympian

...on holiday, white sandy beaches all around and a cocktail in your hand

...happy and healthy, with your friends and family around you

Always looking forward, never backwards, you can promise yourself that you will not be the same person for your experience and in hand with that is the opportunity to really be you.

Wear black if it makes you look good

I like dark colours, only because they are slimming and they generally make me look good.

But if you dress dark because you are down or already mourning an unknown outcome, then you will feel worse.

Use colour to brighten your mood and the moods of those around you, dress according to your personality.

If you feel bright today, be bright, energy and maybe a little fun will follow.

Find a project or creative outlook

During my days off for the first third of my treatment I managed to lay weed mats, shift a ton of gravel, plant some fine banana trees and shift the outdoor furniture to a new deck. The deck was built by somebody else. This project was a great thing for my mind and body to get stuck into; it was a combination of physical exercise and mental challenge that had a great outcome.

These days I don't look at my garden as something to do with my illness, I just enjoy it and love to sit in it during the summer months surrounded by plants that would not otherwise be there.

Find a project, throw yourself into it and dump some of that excess energy, then there won't be enough left to be sad with.

Good things still happen to sick people

Don't expect to win the lotto, but good things can still happen.

Out of the blue I was offered a great job barely two weeks out of treatment, I was honest about my situation and they still wanted to keep me on.

Life is challenging, but I have always stuck to the "everything happens for a reason" explanation.

Doom attracts gloom, it's a natural law, keeping positive and focused might just make a good thing happen.

And besides you never know about the lotto, as they say "it could be you".

Avoid miracle cures

You might be feeling desperate, lost and be looking for any kind of guidance.

Eat well, get some anti oxidants, get your colours into you and listen to your specialists.

If somebody offers you a new and exciting non-medical miracle cure, then it's most likely not going to help. Spend your money on a juicer, or a massage, or a treat for your loved one.

From experience, being sold a couple of expensive bottles of goji berry juice at an expo was not a great investment. I would not question the valuable properties of the juice, but I would question the 'cure all' suggestions that came with it. That was early days with the disease and at a stage when it's easy to believe.

Only join a group if that's your thing

Support groups can be good for some people.

If you think it will help to talk to fellow survivors then go for it; remember that you don't *have* to go if you don't want to.

It's a personal decision, and perhaps one that needs to be made on the day.

You may make new friends with shared experiences, but remember there will probably be doses of sadness involved too.

If travel is difficult or anonymity is preferred there are plenty of support groups with great websites and active forums. Message boards where people, can ask their questions, swap their experiences and share their stories.

A fairly new and great example is easily found at www.LifebloodLIVE.org.nz, where the forum is moderated by haematology nurses and support staff from the Leukaemia & Blood Foundation.

Don't do something out of character

You are still the same person that you were the day before you were sick.

Finding religion or becoming a workaholic to prove a point will not be a good use of energy, focus on being strong and healthy instead.

Some people may find the diversion of a new way of life a good way of dealing with or avoiding the reality of what's happening.

Personally, I like to deal with the stuff that I can understand.

Question:

What's scarier than having the disease?

Answer:

Being told you're clear.

Believe it or not, after all that toxic treatment stress and worry the strangest thing will be coming to terms with having your life back. With all the questions that suddenly come up.

Will it come back? When? Will I be fit again? Who's looking out for me now? How can I plan for the future? How can I commit to a new job?

Concentrate on being happy, enjoy experiences as your sense of tastes and your abilities come back, live, and love living.

Negative energy and stress could be part of the puzzle that makes up the disease, avoid it if you can.

Security blanket

Your security blanket is the health system, when they are there looking out for you.

Scanning you, testing you and treating you.

You may feel pretty grim and sick, but once you are finished with them you may feel lost, suddenly the help and support that you have been taking for granted is suddenly taken away and you feel alone, and abandoned.

Your medical practitioners are still there in the background and will be available to discuss your fears and worry with you. You can learn to live without them. Enjoy your successes and learn to move on.

Remember that charity is
not a four letter word

The infrastructure of the community we live can help you. There are organizations and government bodies that can help, but you have to ask.

Don't be ashamed or afraid, get out there and ask for help, find out what is available. Everybody has slightly different circumstances and will need assistance in different ways, remember that you are very sick and anything that helps to take pressure off your day-to-day routines is a welcome benefit.

It might be help with grocery and house bills, or a paid taxi back home from the hospital.

If you don't ask, you don't get.

Don't be dwelling on should haves

There's no point at all.

The past is past and you are dealing with now.

Dwelling on things you should have done will only make you down.

Maybe that extra insurance payment may have paid off your house, but you didn't take it for a reason back then, and those reasons will not have changed.

You cannot alter those decisions now, so don't spend time and energy worrying about them you have enough to deal with.

Listen to your body, it knows you best

We all have an inbuilt sense of right and wrong, it's called instinct.

Learn to listen to your instinct and respond to it, your body is going to be suffering an enormous chemical assault to fix you; in return you need to respect your body's wishes and act when it commands.

If you get tired – sleep.

If you are still hungry after a meal – eat.

If you are still thirsty – keep drinking fluids.

Don't keep going because you think you need to, invest in your immediate future and build up energy whenever you can.

The regime of pills

My chemotherapy pills didn't come in fancy colours or sugar coating, they weren't chewable or tasted like fruit.

Depending on the various types of treatment a patient will have a schedule of different pills for different days. As soon as you know this plan map it out on a calendar or in a diary as if your life depended on it.

Not only will a pill plan help you stay on top of taking the right pills on the right time, it will also give you a great indicator on progress and count down the days to your last bitter pill to be swallowed.

There are a lot of people
riding on this bus

Welcome to one of those secret societies that exist beneath the day to day world.

You will be very surprised at the people that have experienced first, second or third hand the very same events that you feel overwhelmed by. One of the benefits of talking to such people and sharing your problem is that everybody you know will know of somebody that has been there before you.

There will be a positive story out there to grab and run with, it's all about information that you can refer back to and rely on when things are looking dark.

You might make new friends or it might just make you feel better, either way it's time well spent.

Everything will get worse
before it gets better

This is one rule of life that I have stuck to very early on and it has carried through my school years, and working years, and especially when battling this disease.

Keep in mind that there will be a light at the end of the tunnel, there will be a better day – it just might not be tomorrow.

When a problem or bad time arises it is usually the tip of the proverbial iceberg, you might feel in the doldrums and be physically rock bottom, but you need to keep focused on getting better and stronger one step at a time.

The rest will fall into place.

The ripple effect

This disease is a stone cast into your still waters and just like a stone in a pond it will:

Cause a big and disturbing splash as it lands smack in the middle of your life.

Then create a bunch of fast moving ripples will charge out from the point of impact covering almost every aspect of your life, as the whirlwind of treatment begins.

Then the new ripples will start to slow down and spread out, until, just as you believe that calm is being restored some of the bigger ripples will bounce off the edge of the pool and come back to haunt you.

The disease and treatment is part of life now, what matters most is how we deal with it.

To survive this war, you've got to become the war

This sentiment is echoed in the lines of a famous fictional Buddhist.

You are being treated, you are progressing, you will complete the cycle and believe that one day your specialist will shake your hand and usher you out of the door a healthy individual.

You have to embrace the process and take each day as it comes, learn as much as you can and keep focused on winning your war one, battle at a time.

You don't have to be Rambo, but a little fight goes a long way.

from the author

They say that everybody has at least one book in them, I'm glad that this was mine.

Having spent some of my years dabbling in fiction, short stories, ambitious unfinished novels and unwanted screenplays I finally found a non-fiction subject that gave me some momentum

At the time I was diagnosed I remember buying a text book to give me some guidance, it was the first time I ever cried in a book shop, and I came away wondering where the fun was. It seemed to me that the subject was laden with technical manuals of one sort or another, but I wanted straight and open advice on what may happen, along with tips on how to cope.

I like to think that this book offers just that, and hope that you find something useful in the passages, maybe even raising a smile on the way.

Thanks for taking the time and best wishes for your future.

Richard Armitt, December 2008

KCC